DIY Tips: How to make your own flushable wet wipes at home

A guide on how to make your adult and baby wet wipes at home.

Gladys Emo

Contents

INTRODUCTION

Homemade Wet Wipes

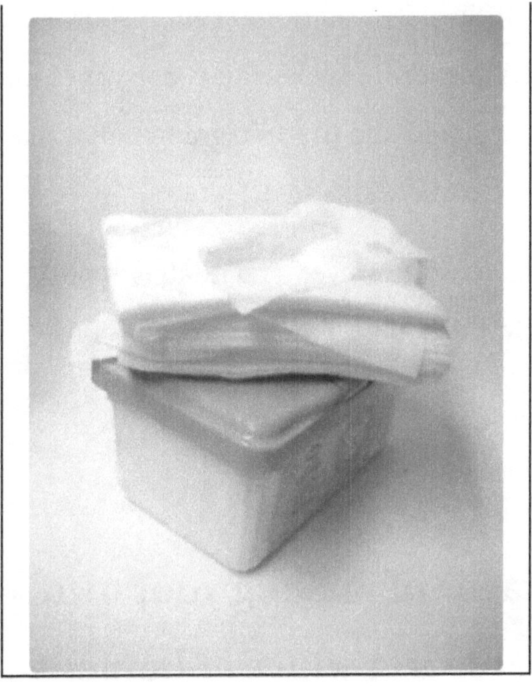

Wet wipes are excellent for wiping your baby and your butt too. Unlike the regular toilet paper, they have you feeling fresh and clean after use. Sadly, they are quite expensive and may cause a strain on your finances if you have to use them continuously. Additionally, a good number of wet wipes manufacturers include ingredients that are harmful and could result in skin irritations around your butt. This is not very pleasant. Again, these wet wipes are in most cases, scented and these fragrances may also irritate adults. No one wants that.

There is good news however and that is, you can make your own flushable wet wipes in your house!

Advantages of making your own flushable wet wipes at home

1. You are in control of the ingredients in your wet wipes, making it as natural as it can possibly be. Also, it is made without plastic, so it can be flushed without fear of getting a clogged sewer.

2. Homemade wipes are cost effective as all materials needed are cheap.

3. You can add this to your list of achievements as a DIY pro!

Disadvantages of making flushable wet wipes at home

1. It takes time

2. It may get messy

3. They may be less effective than the store-bought wet wipes

Making Your Own Flushable Wet Wipes

Ingredients needed:

1. Quality Toilet Paper - Get the best quality you possibly can as it will need to still be together when it has been soaked in water.

2. Distilled Water - Use 350ml of distilled water, or water that has been boiled and cooled down so it is germ free and clean.

3. Coconut Oil - For its antibacterial properties

4. Vinegar Solution - For its antifungal properties

5. Aloe Vera solution

6. Perfume or soap if you would like your wipes to be scented.

Procedure

1. Measure out and cut the length of the tissue you like. Cutting the toilet paper may not be so easy. If you can, make use of an electric knife. Place the cut toilet paper in a bowl

2. In another bowl, pour all liquid ingredients and mix properly

3. Pour the mix into the bowl containing the toilet paper

4. If toilet paper is still in roll, slowly take out the cardboard tube in the middle

5. Pick out wet toilet paper and use as wet wipe.

6. Cover the bowl containing the wet toilet paper to prevent it from getting dry from evaporation

7. It the toilet paper gets dry; you can add some liquid mix to get it wet again.

Other Methods for Homemade Flushable Wet Wipes.

This tutorial is easy to follow.

PREPARATION TIME: 5 minutes

 TIME: 1 minute

TOTAL TIME USED: 6 minutes

DIFFICULTY: Easy

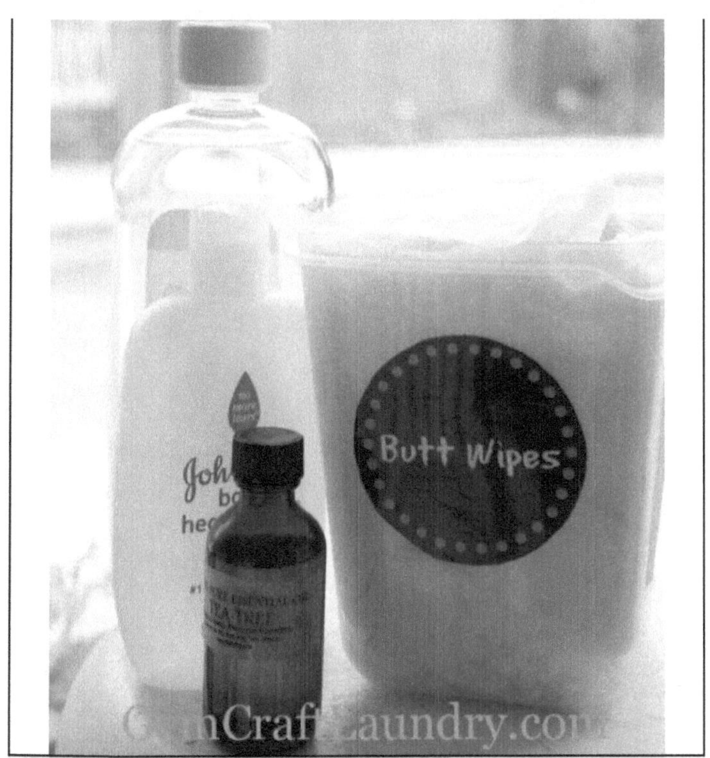

Materials Needed:

- 1 Roll of Paper Towel

- Warm Distilled Water (2 Cups)

- Baby wash

- Coconut oil

- Tea Tree Oil (6-10 drops)

- 1 Air Tight Container

Tools

- A Knife

- Measuring Cup and Measuring spoons

- A Cutting Board

Procedure:

1. Add baby wash, coconut oil and tea tree oil into warm Distilled water in a measuring cup

2. Mix gently

3. Divide the paper towel roll in half. Stand one half upright inside the plastic container.

4. Slowly pour half of the liquid mixture over the paper towels. Flip over the paper towel roll so the drier half is at the top and pour in remaining mixture.

5. Pour the liquid mix slowly on the paper towels. Turn the paper towels over and pour the remaining mix so liquid gets to every part of the towels

6. When the paper towel is well saturated, take out the cardboard tube by pulling it out gently

7. Mark the container and keep in bathroom.

8. Check that your paper towel is not over saturated. Keep some liquid mixture in a spray bottle so you can moisten wipes again if they get dry. The wet paper towel on top should be pulled in its middle to make it easy to pick out when needed

There! Your wet wipes are ready for use!

Another Method for Homemade Flushable Wet Wipes - Kitchen and Household Wipes

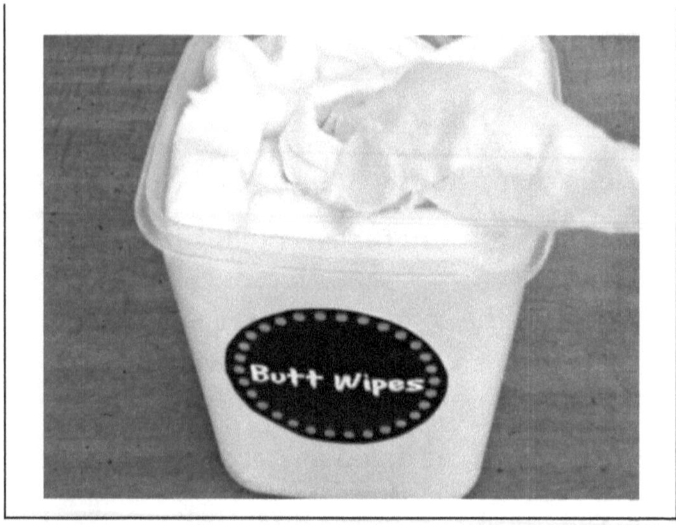

1. Get a paper towel roll of good quality

2 Divide into two by cutting it so you have two short rolls.

3. Take out 15-20 sheets from each of the short rolls and pile them up neatly. This pile will be toilet wipes and the rolls left will be for household or kitchen wipes

4. Use an old toilet wipe container to hold your folded pieces of paper towels

5. Mix 2 tablespoons of vinegar, ¾ cup of water and a couple drops of soap together. You may add a little glycerin if you choose to

6. Pour solution on the folded paper towels and close the lid

7. Your toilet wipes are ready to be kept in the bathroom for use

8. Place the short-reduced rolls of paper towels into a used disinfectant wipes container. If the 15-20 sheets weren't taken out, the rolls would be unable to fit into the container

9. Mix a cup of vinegar, a cup of water and ½ teaspoon of dishwashing soap for each roll

10. Pour solution over the rolls. Allow to sit for six hours approximately

11. Remove the inner cardboard tube by pulling gently

Voila! Two containers of kitchen wipes and one of toilet wipes are now ready for your use.

How to make Homemade Baby Wipes

Now that you have learnt how to make your own wet wipes, below is a guide on how to make your baby wipes.

When you follow this Homemade Baby Wipes Recipe, you will be able to make your own baby wipes at home at a very low cost.

Preparation Time: 5 minutes

Cooking Time: 5 minutes

Total time used: 10 minutes

Ingredients

- 1 **roll of paper towels** cloth-like (I used Bounty brand)
- 2 cups of water
- 2 tablespoons of liquid baby bath soap
- 1 tablespoon of baby oil
- 7 to 8 cups of square or round container

Instructions

1. First, cut the paper towel roll into half using a serrated knife (a bread knife can also work perfectly)

2. Put one part of the halves inside the round or square container. Keep the other half, you can use it later, when you want to make another batch of wipes.

3. Now, boil 2 cups of water for 2 minutes.

4. Then add a little liquid bath soap and baby oil to the boiled water.

5.   If the wipes are wet, they will come out with ease.

6.   Put a lid over the container.

7.   Place the lid over the container securely until you are ready to use it. To use, start by pulling the wipes from the center of the roll, then replace the lid after each use.

8.   Make sure the wipes are kept wet and fresh for up to a week.

9.   In case you have not used all the wipes and they start to dry out, just add some boiled water to refresh the roll.

10.   These baby wipes are not flushable so do not flush them.

Frequently Asked Questions

Q. What are wet wipes?

A: They are cleaning sheets of various kinds—baby wipes, moist toilet tissue, degreasers for industries, make-up cleaners and the likes.

In most cases, they are not flushable in the toilet though they may claim to be. However, as a result of their being unable to be properly broken down in sewerage systems, there is a call to classify all wipes as nonflushable till a standard is agreed on.

Q. What is the problem with wet wipes?

A. Wet wipes need to be firm when wet, so they are stronger that the typical toilet paper. This makes it difficult to break down easily when flushed. As a result, they may block pipes and pumps in sewers.

These wipes can attach themselves to fats in the sewers. They become 'fatbergs' and block pipes. They have to be taken out mechanically and it is very expensive to do that. A lot more problems with blocked sewers is caused by the flushing of non-flushable wipes.

Q. What are wipes made from?

ANS. They are generally made from non-woven materials – usually fibrous materials like cellulose from wood pulp, sometimes reinforced with polymers like viscose. Non-flushable wipes may include man-made fibers like poly(ethylene) or poly(propylene) for extra strength.

Generally, wipes are made of nonwoven fibrous material such as cellulose made from wood pulp. They are sometimes strengthened with viscose or other polymers. Non-flushable wipes may also have artificial fibers like polyethylene or polypropylene as strengtheners. To make a sheet, these fibers are spun into a matted mass and then they are compressed with binders and similar materials.

They can be loaded with sanitary products and preservatives as well as other chemicals, determined by its intended use.

Flushable wipes make use of shorter fibers rather than non-flushable wipes and may also have treatments to enable them break down faster after they've been used.

Q. How are flushable wipes tested?

A. Right now, there is no mandatory test before a product is marked as flushable. Associations like the INDA (US) and EDANA (Europe) have, together with water research bodies worked to create non-mandatory test guidelines for member companies.

These guidelines set out a series of test that products should pass before being marked as flushable. The tests are whether they pass through pipework, whether they clog household or other sewers and how fast its breakdown process is under different water treatment situations.

Q: Does this make it okay to flush wipes that are marketed as flushable?

A. This is not a straightforward situation. The INDA and EDANA may be rigorous, but they are not altogether perfect. Their tests are based on specific behavior patterns of consumers - particular amount of wipes in a specific number of flushes. This includes paper and replicated poo.

If these speculated patterns of use are not followed — like a person using way too many wipes before a flush — the wipes will not disintegrate the anticipated way and this will cause some problems

Another problem is that the guidelines are non-mandatory and also regulated by self. While member companies of the INDA and EDANA may put in the work by testing and improving the flushability of their products, not much can be done to stop any non-member companies from marking random unflushable products as flushable. It is because of this that water companies have asked that every wipe be marked as unflushable until there is an establishment of a general standard for flushability that all companies will be legally bound to comply with.

The fact that there are wipes marked as flushable and others that are not, can cause problems too as users may not know the difference, may not understand the difference or may not be bothered by it. Marking all wipes as non-flushable makes the message simple to consumers, and may help with the problems caused by the flushing of non-flushable wipes.

However, on the manufacturer's end, these products are in demand. There has also been an investment of time and other resources in the development of materials that match the best standards available, in alliance with the water industry, so in order to sell, they will stick to the claims that their wipes are flushable.

Q. Do paper towels cost more than wet wipes?

A. No. In this case, they are bought to make DIY wet wipes. Reusable wipes and kitchen towels are used for most kitchen chores so as to save money and be less wasteful. Also, you have a lot of more homemade wipes for less money than you would for store-bought wipes. If your paper roll comes with 80 paper towels, you will get 160 wet wipes.

The numbers are different depending on the brands and materials you choose to use. In our procedure, we have used only a few drops of tea tree oil so as to avoid the growth of molds or mildew. You can leave out the tea tree oil if you will be making your wipes in small amounts that can be used up in a few days.

This is the way to get wipes that have dried out to be moistened again: Make the toilet wipe solution and spray it on wipes that have dried out.

www.ingramcontent.com/pod-product-compliance
Lightning Source LLC
Chambersburg PA
CBHW051429250726
48655CB00003B/1310